Home Isolation in COVID-19

Table o

Preface ....

Foreword .....

Introduction 8

Abbreviations 11

Story of COVID-19 13

    About COVID-19 13

        Incubation period 13

        Mode of spread 14

        COVID19 care path way - Entry and Exit 15

        Various Symptoms 16

        Warning signs – (Moderate – severe cases) . 16

        Classification of the disease based on severity 17

        Stages of the COVID-19 18

        Phases of COVID-19 20

        Major complications in COVID 22

        Diagnosis of COVID 23

Home Isolation 29

    Items needed to fight against COVID19 in home isolation 31

    Generic precautions 34

    Masks vs Respirators 38

How to reuse masks 41

Home isolation precautions 43

Monitoring COVID-19 patient 46

Diet 58

Treatment 60

Anti- pyretic drugs 60

Anti-viral drugs 60

Anti-biotic drugs 62

Antiparasitic drugs 62

Antacid drugs 63

Anti-inflammatory drugs 63

Anti-coagulants 64

Immune boosters 65

Vaccination 66

References 68

Preface

I am Dr Sai Vani, specialized in Nephrology. I felt apprehended when I heard my father tested COVID-19 positive. He is 67years old with hypertension and diabetes, but he recovered at home with timely monitoring and certain precautions without the need of hospital admission. Though I am a doctor I am worried initially on the day of the result, but we could win in the fight of COVID.

Then, this event inspired me to enlighten the public who do not have awareness and become panic, which makes the things worse in COVID. I want to share my own story to allay the anxiety of most of the people and relieve their fear of COVID.

For this work, I am blessed with wholehearted support from my family, my husband Dr B. Ravindra Babu MS MCh., my mother in law B. Janakamma and my father in law B.Ramakrishna Murthy M Com Retd Lecturer, in taking care of my kids who are small Aarunya 4 year and Shanmukh 1 and a half year old. With the support of my parents Y. Sai Sudhakar Retired

AGM, Y. Satyavathi B com. I could compose and complete this book. My sister Y.Harini MCA, supported me in editing the book.

The dream of writing the book was from my teacher and my mentor Dr Manisha Sahay, Professor and HOD of Nephrology, Osmania Medical College, Hyderabad who always inspires me to write and share the knowledge.

I thank each and every one who supported me to make this accomplish.

Foreword

I have great pleasure in introducing Dr (Mrs.) Sai Vani, consultant nephrologist. She did her DM in Nephrology from Osmania Medical College and General hospital, Hyderabad. She had an excellent academic career and passed her exams in flying colors. She is very sincere and hardworking. Her compassion towards patients is admirable. She was member of the team which performed the first ever simultaneous kidney pancreas transplantation at Osmania General Hospital for a young diabetic patient with kidney failure.

Corona virus disease COVID-19 has spread like wildfire and has affected the lives of people all over the world. Though the disease may be severe in about 15% patients who need hospitalization, almost 85% recover without any specific treatment. These patients do not need admission to hospital. In today's world because of the extreme apprehension among public, many patients are getting admitted to the hospitals even though they do not need admission. On one hand, this leads to non-availability of hospital beds for those patients who really require admission and oxygen. On the other hand, it leads to wasteful expenditure.

Thus, Home isolation is very important and pertinent in today's times. This book is very relevant as it focuses on this burning need. The book highlights the home isolation in detail with all precautions which need to be taken to protect the other family members as well. As the author had personal experience with home isolation, she has brought out all the practical issues as well.

I congratulate Dr Sai Vani for bringing out this excellent and very readable book and wish her all the success.

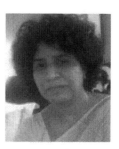

Professor (Dr) Manisha Sahay

Professor and Head, Department of Nephrology

Osmania Medical college & Osmania General Hospital,

Hyderabad Councilor,

International Society of Nephrology (ISN)

Chair, South Asia Regional Board, International Society of Nephrology Editor in Chief, Indian Journal of transplantation (IJT)

Vice President, Indian Society of Nephrology

Fellow Royal College of Physicians (FRCP, London) Fellow Indian Society of Organ Transplantation (FISOT) Fellow, Indian society of Nephrology (FISN)

Committee member, Sister Renal center committee, (ISN-SRC) Committee member, American Nephrologists of Indian origin (ISN ANIO) Executive member, Indian Society of Organ transplant (ISOT)

Introduction

COVID-19 is a novel viral disease started in Wuhan city of China in Dec 2019, which is a highly contagious, airborne spread to 180 countries. Its origin is from the bats, now this pandemic affected every country's social life and economy.

We need not get panic with the news of COVID-19 positive report but should be cautious and watchful. Follow simple tips which help people to isolate or quarantine at home and approach doctor at the needy time so that the right person gets right treatment as the health facilities are meagre compared to the number of affected people.

In this COVID-19 pandemic, only 14% of the affected people require hospitalization, the remaining 86% can be managed at home with the simple treatment. Among those hospitalized, only 2%requires ICU treatments needing respiratory assistance.

Though it is a contagious disease, for me it is a lifestyle disease. People with a good lifestyle, self-disciplined can win the disease effectively.

The **at-risk individuals for severe COVID** are elderly people whose age is greater than 55 years (as age increases the risk of severity increases), kids and other Comorbid persons i.e., with other underlying medical conditions like hypertension, diabetes, cardiovascular disease, chronic lung disease, chronic renal disease, obesity, rheumatologic disease, cancer patients on treatment and Pregnancy.

Each person will have different questions like

- *When do people know that they are infected?*
- *How does it spread?*
- *What is COVID19 care pathway? when is to enter? when is to exit?*
- *What are the symptoms of COVID-19 infected people?*
- *What are the different stages of spread in the community?*
- *How does the disease manifest in an infected person?*
- *What are the different phases inside the body?*
- *What are the major complications?*

Home Isolation in COVID-19

- *Who can be managed at home?*
- *What are the things required for home isolation?*
- *What are the different types of masks?*
- *How to wear the mask properly?*
- *How to remove the mask properly?*
- *Which mask is recommended?*
- *Can we reuse a mask?*
- *Which diet should the infected person follow?*
- *What sort of precautions that care taking person needs to take?*
- *What sort of monitoring is required during isolation?*
- *During which stage, infected person should contact emergency service?*
- *What is the COVID19 monitoring calendar?*
- *Is there any post exposure prophylaxis?*
- *As of now, what is the status of vaccination?*

This book answers these questions.

Abbreviations

SOB	Shortness of breath
Ct	Cycle threshold
CTSS	Computerized Tomogram Severity Score
CO-RADS	COVID19 – Radiological and Data based system
CT Scan	Computerized Tomogram
Tab	Tablets
Inj	Injection
SpO2	Peripheral capillary oxygen saturation
PR	Pulse Rate
PI	Pulsatility index
RT PCR	Reverse transcriptase polymerase chain reaction
True-NAT	Chip based Nucleic acid test
CB-NAAT	Cartridge based nucleic acid amplification system
ELISA	Enzyme Linked Immunosorbant Assay
CLIA	Chemi Luminescent Immuno Assay
MMR	Measles Mumps Rubella

| BCG | Bacillus Calmette Geurine |

Story of COVID-19

We can manage many of the COVID-19 persons at home, with Positive attitude, moral boost and support from "**Local active Emergency Medical Team**" and necessary lab. By watchful monitoring of symptoms and signs periodically with necessary investigations once in every 4th day, with guidance from local doctor we can manage at home. This will help hospitals to allot beds to the needy at right time. Please note that "**Only mild cases can be maintained under home isolation**".

Let us understand Incubation period, mode of spread, symptoms, different stages in COVID transmission, different phases of the COVID disease and its diagnosis. We will be discussing isolation and quarantine after that.

About COVID-19

Incubation period

The duration between exposure to COVID19 person and appearance of the symptoms, is on an average 5- 6 days but can occur up to 14 days. The infected person is infective even in pre symptomatic period, 1-3 days prior to onset of the symptoms.

Mode of spread

COVID-19 is highly **contagious** disease, based on the current evidence; the COVID-19 virus is transmitted between people through droplets, fomites and close contact, with possible spread through feces. It is not merely airborne.

Whenever the infected person coughs, sneezes or talks, the droplets fall on the surface within a distance of 6 feet. When the normal person comes in close contact with infected person, without wearing the mask or touch the surface with droplets and again touches the face, the virus enters the body through mouth, nose or eyes.

Frequent hand washing, wearing the mask and face shield and maintaining physical distance helps to prevent this.

Home Isolation in COVID-19

COVID19 care path way - Entry and Exit

Entry

A person enters the COVID-19 care pathway after s/he is *screened,* based on a standardized case definition, including assessment of symptoms, and meets criteria for a suspect case.

- **Suspect cases** - "persons or patients under investigation" (PUIs) in some contexts.

- **Probable cases** - suspected cases with testing for SARS-CoV-2 is inconclusive or not available.

- **Confirmed cases** -   persons with laboratory confirmation of COVID-19.

EXIT

Discontinue transmission-based precautions (including isolation)

- **For symptomatic patients**: 10 days after symptom onset, plus at least 3 days without symptoms (without fever and respiratory symptoms).

- **For asymptomatic patients:** 10 days after testing positive.

Various Symptoms

Fever or chills, sore throat, dry cough, new loss of smell or taste, diarrhea, fatigue, muscle pains in mild cases.

Loss of smell or taste indicates good prognosis in the disease progression.

Warning signs – (Moderate – severe cases)

Seek emergency hospital admission in case of below warning signs.

COVID-19 person with shortness of breath, pressure in the chest, new confusion, unconsciousness and bluish lips, should seek emergency medical help.

Classification of the disease based on severity

The COVID19 disease can be classified according to the symptoms and signs into mild, moderate, severe and critical disease.

Home Isolation in COVID-19

	Mild	Moderate	Severe
Symptoms	Fever, cough, cold, body pains, loss of smell and taste, diarrhea	Chest pain, Shortness of breath	Altered sensorium, Shortness of breath
Respiratory rate	<24 / min	24 – 30/min	> 30/min
Pulse rate	60 – 100/min	>100/min	>100/min
SPO2 (Blood oxygen saturation level)	>94% in room-air	90 – 94% in room-air	<90 % in room-air

CT Severity Score	< 9 /25	9 – 15/25	15 – 25/25

Critical illness: The person may have septic shock or multi organ dysfunction or Acute Respiratory Distress Syndrome (ARDS).

Critical illness with cytokine storm: Critically ill person with CRP>100mg/dl, Ferritin >900mg/dl, D dimer>1500 micro gram/liter

Only mild cases can be maintained under home isolation

Stages of the COVID-19

The rapidity in the spread of COVID19 within the community depends on the stages of the disease. The source of contact can be traced in initial stages but in later stages of community spread, the source cannot be traced. Multiple clusters are affected later causing epidemic.

Home Isolation in COVID-19

Stage 1	Cases of infected people	Infected people are **imported** from affected countries.
Stage 2	Local transmission	The source of the infected person(person with travel history from affected countries), is known and can be located.
Stage 3	Community transmission	This takes place when the source of infection can't be traced and isolated.
Stage 4	Epidemic	Multiple clusters are involved

Now this is a **Pandemic** disease involving more than 180 countries

Home Isolation in COVID-19

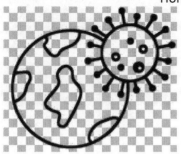

Phases of COVID-19

The COVID-19 person passes through three phases – in two-week period.

Initially, in the first week viral response occurs and declines at the end of the first week, in the second week host immune response increases resulting in pulmonary and hyper inflammatory phases.

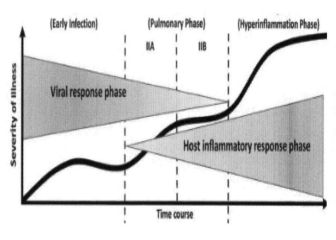

There are 3 main phases:

1. Phase 1 - Early infection phase
2. Phase 2 - The Pulmonary phase
3. Phase 3 - Hyper inflammatory phase

Early infection phase

This is the first stage of COVID-19. The symptoms in this phase are:

- The virus multiplies inside the body and causes mild symptoms.
- Investigations show Lymphopenia

Anti-viral medication is helpful at this phase

The Pulmonary phase

This is the second phase of COVID-19. This phase can be divided into two.

2a) Shortness of breath (SOB)

2b) fall of oxygen saturations – It's better to hospitalize in this situation

The characteristics of this phase:

- The immune system is strongly affected by infection.
- Respiratory symptoms can be observed
- Cough, shortness of breath, low oxygen saturation levels
- Chest imaging shows abnormality.

Antivirals and steroids are helpful in this phase.

Hyper inflammatory phase

This is the third phase of COVID-19.

Activated immune system causes injury to heart, kidneys and other own organs. The inflammatory cytokines release may be more, ten times their normal levels causing cytokine storm – which is lethal, causes damage to all organs with thrombosis of the blood vessels and hampers the blood supply.

Steroids, Plasma therapy and Tocilizumab are helpful in this phase.

Major complications in COVID
Happy hypoxia

The uniqueness of this disease is, though the oxygen saturations fall, the patients do not experience any symptom, they collapse suddenly. This can be avoided by periodic monitoring with pulse oximeter.

Disseminated intravascular thrombosis

It causes decreased blood supply to the organs causing multi organ dysfunction and death.

It can be diagnosed by monitoring '**Inflammatory markers**' and '**D-dimer**' in COVID profile.

Diagnosis of COVID

There are two types of tests – Serological and Molecular

Serological tests:

The antibodies inside the plasma of an infected person are tested.

Their quantification helps to decide the donor for plasma donation.

Molecular tests:

Here molecular antigen (specific genetic material of the virus) is tested;

Sample is taken from the mouth or naso pharynx and dipped into the solution which inactivates the virus.

Antigen kit tests: The antigen is not amplified. **True NAT, CB NAAT and COVID RT PCR:** The antigen is amplified, so more sensitive.

Radiology

Chest X ray and CT scan chest

Table: Diagnostic test and its importance

Diagnostic test	Importance
Serological tests	**Methods - ELISA and CLIA** This test measures the amount of antibodies or proteins present in the blood Not useful for diagnosis, only for surveillance.

Become positive in 30% of patients in first week, 50% in second week and 70% in third week of infection.

Indicates whether the person is infected in the past or not.

IgM antibody – First antibodies to appear inside the infected person, indicates the person is recently infected with in 1 week.

IgG antibody – appear during IgM antibodies declining phase and more specific antibodies to the virus, indicates the person is infected in the past two weeks.

Antibody kit test	This test is not for diagnosis, only to know the immunity for surveillance purposes.

Molecular tests	Genetic Material (antigen) tested Sample is taken from the mouth or naso pharynx and dipped into the solution which inactivates the virus. positive only during the infection
Antigen kit test	Antigen is not amplified. If the test result is positive it confirms, the negative result does not rule out COVID.
True NAT	Molecular antigen is amplified, so more sensitive and easily portable, can be taken to containment areas. Chip based nucleic acid test. The report can be given at the earliest.

CBNAAT	Cartridge based Nucleic acid amplification test
	Initially used in TB, similar to True NAT but not portable.
COVID PCR	This test is highly sensitive.
	high Ct values indicate low viral load
	Low Ct values indicate high viral load
Chest X ray	Changes in the lungs are found at late phase.
	Shows peripheral ground glass opacities.
CT chest	More sensitive than chest X ray
	Sometimes COVID PCR may be negative but symptomatic patients can be diagnosed by CT chest, CO-

Home Isolation in COVID-19

RAD score indicates the disease, CTSS indicates the severity of the disease.

Home Isolation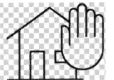

The decision as to whether to isolate and care for an infected person at home depends:

1) **Clinical evaluation of the COVID-19 patient** – only in mild cases after evaluating the person without the comorbidities as described in the previous text.
2) **Evaluation of the home setting** - Preferably individual homes with well-ventilated with possibility of implementation of infection prevention control.
3) **The ability to monitor the clinical evolution of a person with COVID-19 at home** – The care taker should monitor the COVID19 person properly and should know when to seek the medical advice.

Let us understand what the difference between Isolation and Quarantine is.

Isolation: Separating the person who is COVID-19 tested positive, without comorbidities

Home Isolation in COVID-19

and asymptomatic for 10 days, with comorbidities for 20 days.

Quarantine: Separating the person who is exposed to the COVID-19, from last day of exposure to 14 days. During this period be watchful for symptoms of COVID.

If any symptoms are experienced during quarantine period, please consult the doctor and get tested for COVID-19.

Home Isolation in COVID-19

Items needed to fight against COVID19 in home isolation

Let us know what all items required for home isolation.

1) **Mask**:

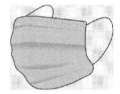

Cloth mask, surgical mask, three layered surgical mask, N95 mask (Respirator).

2) **Disinfectants:**

Read the directions to use properly - use sites for the disinfectant, precautionary statements and contact time.

Keep them away from kids with lids tightly closed.

3) **Disposable gloves**:

Home Isolation in COVID-19

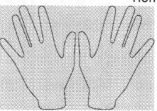

The care taker of the COVID19 person should wear disposable gloves while serving the person and cleaning the toilets after use by COVID-19 person, washing the clothes of COVID-19.

Throw the gloves in closed covered dustbin, after removal of the gloves wash the hands thoroughly.

4) **Face shield**:

The COVID-19 person and his care taker both should wear mask and face shield whenever they come in contact.

5) **Thermometer**:

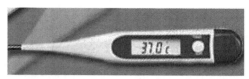

Home Isolation in COVID-19

2 in number, one to check the temperature of the COVID19 person, second one to check the temperature of other persons in the family.

6) **Glucometer**:

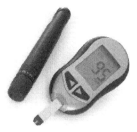

If the infected person is diabetic, RBS should be monitored morning and evening.

7) **Digital BP apparatus**:

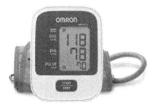

If the infected person is hypertensive, if other family members are also hypertensive use another BP apparatus.

8) **Spirometer**:

Home Isolation in COVID-19

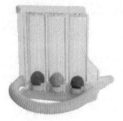

Useful to improve the capacity of lungs.

9) **Pulse oximeter**:

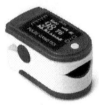

To Monitor Pulse rate, Pulsatility index, Saturations.

Generic precautions

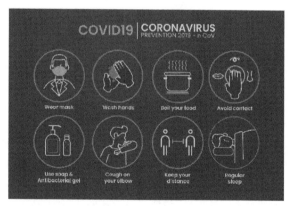

Home Isolation in COVID-19

Below are three golden rules:

1. Hand wash
2. Wearing mask and
3. Physical distancing

Hand wash

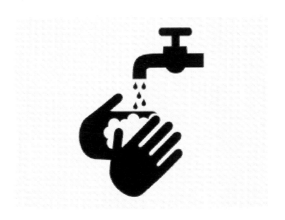

- Frequent hand wash with soap for 20 seconds (singing a happy birthday song) involving front, back of the hands including nails.
- When you are outside, use sanitizer (70% alcohol) to clean your hands after touching the external surfaces.

In general, we suggest washing hands during below conditions

- o   Before eating or preparing food
- o   Before touching face
- o   After using the restroom
- o   After leaving a public place
- o   After blowing nose, coughing, or sneezing
- o   After handling mask
- o   After caring for COVID-19 person

Wearing the mask

Properly fitted mask, covering the mouth and nose properly prevent the aerosol spread into mouth and nose.

Health care workers and care takers of COVID19 person should wear N95 mask (which filters 95% of air droplets). The person who is taking care of COVID-19 also should wear N95 mask covering mouth and nose in Toto.

Home Isolation in COVID-19
How to handle masks

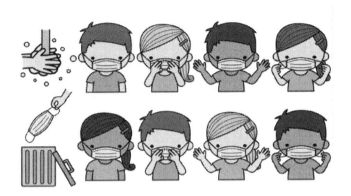

Follow below steps while wearing and removing the mask:

1. Wash hands with soap and water before putting on a mask
2. Mask should cover mouth, nose and chin, make sure there are no gaps between the face and mask
3. Pinch the metal strip, so that it presses gently on nose bridge
4. Remove mask by holding ear loops only
5. Avoid touching the mask while using it
6. Throw the used mask into dust bin. Please do not re-use single-use masks

Masks vs Respirators

There are various kinds of Masks and Respirators available in the market. Below table helps us to decide on Masks and Respirators.

Masks	Respirators
Filters the particles produced from the wearers, when they exit.	Filters the particles that enters and that exits, from the wearers.
One-way protection	Two-way protection
Loosely fit	Tightly fit to the face otherwise not effective
Cloth masks, Surgical masks- single layer, triple layer	N 95(US), FFP2(EN), P2(EN),KN95(Chinese) Usually used in health care and care takers of COVID

Home Isolation in COVID-19

There are two varieties of Respirators

1. Valved Respirators
2. Non Valved Respirators

Below table helps us to determine, Which Respirators are suggestible to use:

Valved Respirators	Non Valved Respirators
Easier to exhale air, no moist builds.	The exhaled air accumulates, so fog appears
Exhaled air is not filtered	Exhaled and inhaled air both are filtered
Should not be used by COVID patients as the surrounding people are at risk	Useful for COVID patients
Useful in Construction workers	Surrounding people are not at risk

There are different types of Respirators available in the market based on percentage of 0.3 micron or above size Particles filtered. Below table lists

39

different types of respirators available in different countries based on their filter level.

Percentage of 0.3 micron or above size Particles filtered	NIOSH part of CDC (American standards)	Filtering Face Piece (European Standards) 149/2001 –FFP series, 143-Pseries	Chinese / Korean Standards
80 %		FFP1,P1	
94% - 95%	N 95 (95%)	FFP2 (94%), P2(94%)	KN95
99%	N 99	FFP3(99%)	

99 -100%	N 100 (99.7%)	P3(99.95 %)	

How to reuse masks

Cloth Masks

Keep the cloth masks in diluted bleach used in household settings for 5 minutes, wash them and dry them under sunlight.

Surgical masks (Single layer, triple layer)

Surgical masks should not be reused.

N95, FFP2, P2 (Respirators)

N95 masks should not be washed only kept in sunlight.

The N95 masks should be 5 in number for each person they should write name and number on each, use daily one for 5 days and alternate accordingly, day by day up to 1 month

Never use the masks with the valves.

Physical distancing

Home Isolation in COVID-19

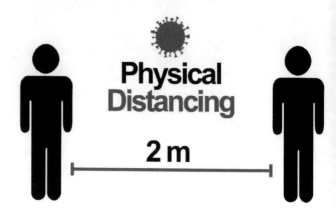

- **Inside the home:**
    - Avoid close contact with people who are sick.
    - If possible, maintain 6 feet distance between the person who is sick and other household members.
- **Outside the home:**
    - Maintain at least 6 feet of distance between yourself and others (people who don't live in your household).
    - Try to avoid gatherings.
    - Work from home if feasible
    - Stay home stay safe unless emergency demands

Home Isolation in COVID-19

- Hold meetings online
- Avoid public transport
- Use Phones for chatting

Home isolation precautions

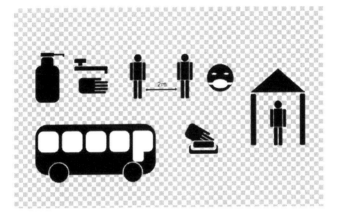

One should follow below steps in home isolation process.

1. Isolate COVID-19 person, in a separate room with attached bathroom. If not available, provide them a separate well-ventilated room. After each usage of toilet ask them to pour disinfectant. The next person using the same toilet should wait for '***contact time***' of disinfectant. Next person should wear gloves

and mask, clean the toilet, handles and taps with soap water and later with the disinfectant.

2. **Quarantine** other household members who are at risk for severe COVID illness like elder people - age more than 55 (as age increases risk of severity of the illness increases), pregnancy and children, underlying medical conditions as explained earlier in this text into other separate room.

3. Dedicate essentially one person for **serving isolated** person preferably young without the comorbidities. Going further we will refer this person as '**care taker**' in this book.

4. It is better to avoid entering isolated room. Wear disposable gloves while cleaning the isolated room, pre clean the surface with soap and water (reduces the germs) later apply disinfectants (kills germs) with appropriate contact time, wash hands with soap and water after throwing the gloves into closed and covered disposable bin.

5. Clean all frequently touch surfaces like tables, door knobs, light switches, handles, phones, keyboards, toilets, faucets, sinks.

Home Isolation in COVID-19

6. Please note that, diluted house hold bleach with contact time of 1 minute can also be used as disinfectant.

7. Separate the clothes, towels, plates and glasses, other utensils for isolated person use. If isolated person is stable, s/he should do his/her own work. If they are sick, the care taker should take care of isolated persons with all precautions.

8. Wash the isolated person clothes separately, in machine at 60 -90degree centigrade, if machine is not present the linen should be soaked in bleach for 30min. Later wash and dry in sunlight.

9. Care taker should wear mask preferably N95, face shield and disposable gloves, maintain physical distance while serving COVID-19 person.

10. COVID-19 person should wear N95mask, face shield when they come in close contact to the care taker or other house hold members.

11. Follow cough etiquette by all.

12. Daily **steam inhalation** thrice and **betadine** gargling has shown some benefit

Home Isolation in COVID-19

13. Take the contact number of local volunteer or emergency medical team to contact or Local doctor and keep it handy for emergency.

14. Take a calendar and note the day of symptom onset and watch daily as more complications between 8th and 12th day of symptom onset.

15. Watch for symptoms of COVID-19 in other household members and care taker in 2 - 14 days, if present get tested.

Monitoring COVID-19 patient

In COVID-19 disease, only 14% patients require hospital admission other 86% can be recovered at home by following home isolation tips mentioned in this book. Along with this, we should be watchful to determine, when the person requires admission which is possible by careful monitoring of the COVID-19 person by care taker.

Usual monitoring at home

1. Daily check for the new onset of symptoms and watch for warning signs mentioned Warning signs – (Moderate – severe cases). if present call emergency medical service and admit them in the hospital

Home Isolation in COVID-19

2. If the COVID person is diabetic or hypertensive, record Blood pressure and Random blood sugar twice a day daily. Maintain Blood pressure of 130/80 and Fasting blood sugar of <110mg/dl, post prandial blood sugar >140mg/dl, Random blood sugar 110 to 140mg/dl. **If readings are not in the range, consult treating physician through tele consultation.**

3. Daily monitor temperature with digital thermometer, thrice a day whenever symptoms are observed.

4. Every 6 hourly check Pulse rate (PR - Normal value 60-100), SPO2 (saturation of blood with oxygen, Normal value above 95%) before and after normal walking for 6 minutes, Pulsatility index (indicates peripheral blood supply to the fingers 0.02% to 20%) through Pulse oximeter. **If saturation falls below 95% or after walk if saturation falls below 5% of the previous value, it's a danger sign contact emergency service system immediately**.

5. **Respiratory rate** (RR): Observe the affected person without informing him/her how many breaths s/he is taking in 15sec and multiply it by 4 if it is **more than 24** it indicates warning sign. If it **increases more than 30** it is definitely the emergency. Activate emergency medical system immediately.

Maneuvers to increase lung capacity

1. **Spirometer**: Take spirometer first exhale fully and keep mouth piece of the spirometer inside the mouth and try to inflate and rise the balls in the spirometer and wait for 5sec and release, reverse it take full inspiration, exhale and wait for 5 sec, ,do 10 times each session 4 times a day, preferably before meal and before going to bed. It increases the lung capacity.

2. Maintaining **prone** position most of the time increases the lung capacity.

3. **Yoga** – pranayama containing Anulom-Vilom, Bhramari, Kapalbhati and Bhastrika.

Home Isolation in COVID-19

Investigational Monitoring (COVID Profile)

Investigations should be repeated every 4 days after diagnosis of COVID or from the onset of symptoms.

Complete Blood Picture and Erythrocyte Sedimentation Rate (CBP and ESR):

1. CBP shows Hemoglobin – Indicates anemia,
2. White blood cell count – Increase in total count indicates secondary infection,
3. Decrease in Lymphocyte count – suggests COVID infection, if it falls less than 1000 indicates severity, zero lymphocyte syndrome indicates severity
4. Absent Eosinophil count – suggests COVID-19
5. Platelet count- decrease indicates the severity, may progress to Disseminated Intravascular Coagulation (DIC)

Renal Function Test (RFT): Indicates how kidneys are affected with the COVID

Liver Function Test (LFT): Indicates how Liver is affected with the COVID

RFT and LFT helps in the prescription of drugs.

Inflammatory Markers:

CRP (< 10mg/L): High levels can be seen in the inflammatory disorder, malignancy, CAD and obesity, etc.

Serum Ferritin (12 – 300 ng/ml for male, 12 – 150 ng/ml for female): High levels can be seen in inflammatory conditions, infections, malignancy and chronic alcoholism.

LDH (Lactate dehydrogenase)-125 – 220(2yrs to 12yrs),180 – 300(>12yrs) u/l – inflammatory marker, indicates ongoing inflammation

IL6 interleukin6 (5 – 15 PG/ml)
Normal concentration of IL6 does not exclude the possibility of an ongoing inflammatory process.

D – Dimer (< 0.50µg/ml) It is increased in coagulopathy, malignancy, pregnancy, CLD and with increasing age, etc. progressive increasing of D-Dimer is a bad prognostic indicator

Procalcitonin - normal level (0.10 – 0.49 ng/ml) Normal levels are usually found in COVID-19 infection, elevated levels suggest bacterial infection.

Cytokine storm: occurs in phase3

Cytokine storm is indicated by exponential rise of inflammatory markers

Marker	Cytokine storm indicator
IL – 6	> 10 times the upper limit (>16 pg/mL
Ferritin	> doubling within 24 hours, > 900 micro g/L at presentation
Lactate dehydrogenase (LDH)	> 250 U/L
C reactive protein (CRP)	High levels (>100 mg/L)
D dimer	Elevated (>1.5 mg/L)

Chest imaging

Chest X-ray:

Ground glass opacities at periphery of lung fields, usually present at advanced condition

CT scan chest:

Two scores

CORADS score – indicates whether the disease is COVID or not no way related to severity, by seeing the score on CT Report need not be panic.

CO – RADS	Level of suspicion	CT Findings
CO-RADS 1	No	normal or non-infectious abnormalities
CO-RADS 2	Low	abnormalities consistent with infections other than COVID-19

CO-RADS 3	Indeterminate	unclear whether COVID-19 is present
CO-RADS 4	High	Abnormalities suspicious for COVID-19
CO-RADS 5	Very high	typical COVID-19
CO-RADS 6	PCR positive	

CT Severity Score-

It indicates severity.

The lungs are divided into 5 lobes, 3 in right, 2 in left, each lobe has given 5 points depending on the severity.

Score in each lobe

1	< 5% of area involved
2	5 – 25% of area involved
3	25 -50% of area involved
4	50 – 75% of area involved
5	>75% of area involved

This score is applied for all 5 lobes of two lungs, and CTSS is calculated

Depending on the total score severity graded

Mild	<9/25
Moderate	9 – 15/25
Severe	>15/25

Home Isolation in COVID-19

Monitoring Calendar

Day (Symptom onset, test given)	Date	Daily PR, SPO2 – 4 hrly Respiratory rate – 12 hrly RBS, BP – 12 hrly Spirometry – 4 sessions, Each session 10 times Yoga – pranayama – 12 hrly	Investigations (COVID profile) Every 4th day
Day 1			
Day 2			

Home Isolation in COVID-19

Day3			
Day4			COVID profile
Day5			
Day6			
Day7			
Day8 Most complicatio ns			COVID profile
Day9			
Day10			
Day11			
Day12			COVID profile
Day13			

Day14

Diet

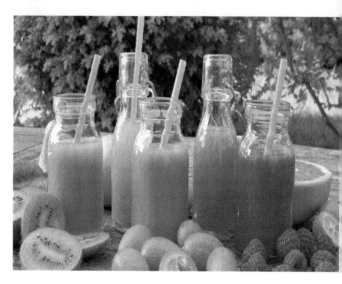

COVID-19 patient should incorporate below diet in their daily routine.

Increase hydration

The disease is hyper catabolic. Daily 3-4 liters of liquid diet is required, as water loss is more from the body. This liquid diet will help in increasing the liquidity of the blood preventing thrombotic tendency.

Increase protein intake

As the disease is hyper catabolic (increased protein breakdown) the requirement of protein increases. One cup of pulses in the morning and evening or 2egg whites in the morning and evening to be taken.

Immune boosters

Vitamin C – The foods rich in vitamin C are Guava, Pineapple, Oranges, Lemon, Amla should be taken.

Vitamin D – Milk or stay in sunlight for 1hour daily

Zinc- Zinc rich foods are pulses, dry fruits.

Home Isolation in COVID-19

Treatment

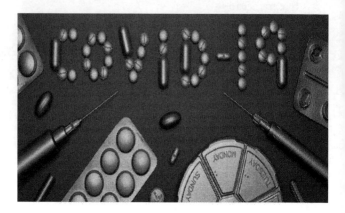

Please find below suggested treatment for COVID-19. Mostly symptomatic treatment is sufficient for home isolation except in special situations.

Anti- pyretic drugs

Tab paracetamol 500mg thrice or four times a day, in case of fever

Anti-viral drugs

Favipiravir (200mg tablets) –

9 tablets in the morning and 9 in the evening with 12 hours gap for first day, followed

Home Isolation in COVID-19

by 4 tablets in the morning and 4 tablets in the evening for 10 days.

It is not necessary for all, it decreases the viral load, which decreases the after effects of inflammatory phase.

It is given to the patients with continuous fever, age >55 years, other medical illness like (Hypertension, Diabetes, CKD, COPD, CVD, Cancer patients, Rheumatologic diseases) or >two inflammatory markers rise in COVID profile more than 2 times or lymphocyte count <1000 or lymphocyte zero syndrome which indicates the severity

Renal disease patients, liver disease patients should take on doctor's advice.

Remdesivir Injection –

should be used in initial viremic phase in moderate to severe cases in the hospital.

Anti-biotic drugs

Not to be given routinely, only in case of signs of secondary bacterial infections (rise in WBC count, rise in procalcitonin).

Tablets	Dosage	Comments
Doxycycline 100 mg	twice a day for 5 days	Acidity
Azithromycin 500mg	once a day for 5 days	Acidity

Not needed if CBP is normal.

Antiparasitic drugs

Tablets	Dosage	Comments
Ivermectin 12 mg	for 2 days	decreases viral entry, prevents strongyloides stercoralis hyper infection

Please note that this should not be given to kids under 5 years of age

Antacid drugs

To decrease the acidity because of all the above medication they are to be used

Tablets	Dosage	Comments
Pantop 40mg	Once a day	

Ranitidine 150mg	Twice a day	
Famotidine 20mg	Thrice a day	mast cell stabilizer helpful in addition in cytokine release.

Anti-inflammatory drugs

Colchicine –

0.5mg twice a day for 5 days

Prevents the release of cytokines from inflammatory cells.

Steroids

To be used only if saturations fall below 95% or >two inflammatory markers rise in COVID profile more than 2 times the normal, if COVID profile totally could not be done because of financial constraints at least CRP>20mg/dl or lymphocyte count <1000 or lymphocyte zero syndrome which indicates the severity.

Helps to decrease the cytokine release, helpful in the second stage of the disease.

Tablets	**Dosage**

dexamethasone 6mg	Twice a day for 5 days
Prednisolone 40mg	Once a day
methyl prednisolone 8mg	Twice a day

Tab dexamethasone 6mg twice a day for 5 days.

Tab Prednisolone 40mg

Tab methyl prednisolone 8mg twice a day

Anti-coagulants

The main complication of COVID is thrombosis of blood vessels in second phase of the disease.

To prevent this, Inj Heparin 5000units Subcutaneous (SC) thrice a day or Inj Clexane 40microgram SC twice a day.

Injections	Dosage
Heparin 5000 units Subcutaneous (SC)	Thrice a day
Clexane 40microgram SC	Twice a day

They are to be started when D-dimer levels 2-3 times normal or coagulation profile >2 parameters elevated >2 times.

Home Isolation in COVID-19

Immune boosters

Tablets	Dosage
Vitamin C - 1000mg	Twice a day
Zinc 15mg	Twice a day
Vitamin D – 60,000units	Once a week

Post Exposure Prophylaxis: Initially Hydroxychloroquine prescribed for prophylaxis but now the recent studies showed no role.

There is no prophylaxis as of now of proven value in COVID19.

Vaccination

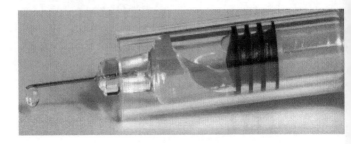

Some studies showed BCG and MMR booster vaccination have protection against COVID19.

COVID19 vaccine is nothing but boosting the immunity with inactivated COVID19 which has antigenicity to produce protective antibodies.

Except Russia all are under trial

In India - Bharath biomedical company's COVID vaccine is in Phase 3 trial.

In Russia Vaccine Sputnik v vaccine is released, started to give to health care workers and teachers.

In England – Oxford AstraZeneca vaccine in phase 3 trial

Home Isolation in COVID-19

In United States – The 6 vaccines are under trial

References

1. Guan WJ, Ni ZY, Hu Y, et al. Clinical Characteristics of Coronavirus Disease 2019 in China. *N Engl J Med* 2020;382:1708-20.

2. Li Q, Guan X, Wu P, et al. Early Transmission Dynamics in Wuhan, China, of Novel Coronavirus-Infected Pneumonia. *N Engl J Med* 2020;382:1199-207.

3. Lauer SA, Grantz KH, Bi Q, et al. The Incubation Period of Coronavirus Disease 2019 (COVID-19) From Publicly Reported Confirmed Cases: Estimation and Application. *Ann Intern Med* 2020.

4. Macgregor H, Hrynick T. COVID-19: Strategies to support home and community-based care. Social Science in Humanitarian Action Platform: 2020

5. World Health Organization. Clinical management of COVID-19: interim guidance. Geneva: World Health Organization; 2020

6. World Health Organization. Home care for patients with Middle East respiratory syndrome coronavirus (MERS-CoV) infection presenting with mild symptoms and management of contacts: interim guidance. Geneva: World Health Organization; 2018

7. World Health Organization. Infection prevention and control during health care for probable or confirmed cases of Middle East respiratory syndrome coronavirus (MERS-CoV) infection: interim guidance. Geneva: World Health Organization; 2019.

8. https://www.ncbi.nlm.nih.gov/pmc/articles/PMC7211650/

9. https://www.ncbi.nlm.nih.gov/pmc/articles/PMC7129451/

10. https://www.ncbi.nlm.nih.gov/pmc/articles/PMC7306198/

11. https://wwwnc.cdc.gov/eid/article/26/8/20-1477_article

12. https://www.tandfonline.com/doi/full/10.1080/22221751.2020.1770129

13. https://fastlifehacks.com/category/home

Home Isolation in COVID-19

Manufactured by Amazon.ca
Bolton, ON

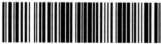